Sex & Tarot

Sex & Tarot

By
Toni Allen

Copyright © 2012, Toni Allen

All rights reserved. No part of this book may be reproduced, stored, or transmitted by any means—whether auditory, graphic, mechanical, or electronic—without written permission of both publisher and author, except in the case of brief excerpts used in critical articles and reviews. Unauthorized reproduction of any part of this work is illegal and is punishable by law.

ISBN 978-1-105975-608

Contents

Introduction 1
   Let's Start at Basics 3
      Suit of Batons and sex in tarot 3
   Now the Emotions get Involved 13
      Tarot suit of Cups and sex in tarot. 13
   Sexual Values 23
      Tarot suit of Coins and sex in tarot 23
   Mind Games & Intellectual Pursuits 33
      Tarot suit of Swords and sex in tarot 33
   The Major Cards and Sex 45
      Card Combinations and practical examples. ... 57
      Infidelity 58
      Jealousy 61
      The Dating Game 63
      Final Thoughts 67

Introduction

My name is Toni Allen and I have been a professional tarot card reader for nearly 30 years. I am now about to share my secrets with you. I am about to divulge information that is rarely written about and barely spoken about. The secret of how to interpret the tarot cards in connection with sex.

During my long career I have done thousands of readings, yes, thousands, and this has given me a wealth of experience and practical knowledge of tarot as a working tool. I use tarot to help guide my clients, help solve their problems, receive messages from loved ones who have passed over, and to explore past lives. I have read for people from all walks of life, from the very rich to the very poor, and there is one subject that makes 99% of them drop their jaw in astonishment when I have dared mention the taboo word during a tarot consultation. Sex.

Yes, sex. Most of us do it, most of us have done it, and yet most of us feel that this most private and personal of pass-times is not something that the tarot cards would ever consider mentioning. Well, now I am going to share a big secret with you. Tarot is all about life as a whole, about human beings as a whole, and therefore, includes…sex. Furthermore, because tarot can see beyond the shallow façade of ego, nothing is private, and it will delve into all of those taboo places that we like to shy away from. You cannot hide from tarot, it will see what you are up to, whether you like it or not.

During a reading people often start to blush, giggle or fiddle when I mention details about their sex activity. All aspects of our lives are important, and often there is little point in discussing a relationship problem and then getting shy over sexual detail if, in fact, the nub of that problem relates to our sex life with our partner. Women ask for guidance on fertility issues; but when I say, "The cards suggest you and your husband are not making enough special time for sex," they look at me dumbfounded, as if the baby will miraculously appear from Heaven above. Men discuss business and money and wanting children, but if I say, "Your wife is unhappy, you're so busy working that you rarely find quality time for sex," they gape and mutter something like, "If I don't find time to satisfy her do you think she'll have an affair?" The answer is generally, "Yes." Sex is important in any loving relationship.

Of course, not all sex takes place in the confines of a 'relationship,' so we'll also be looking at attraction, seduction, romance and what type of person you might be tumbling into bed with on that hot first date. I am not here to titillate, but to offer the true student of tarot my wealth of insight and knowledge of how various sexual problems, issues and dilemmas can be indicated in a tarot reading. Having said that some of my students love this side of tarot and have a hoot when discussing it... I really can't imagine why!

Always remember that a tarot reading is not just one card but an entire inter-relation of all the cards on the table. Unless, of course, you are taking just one card to answer a question. Also take into consideration that all of the examples below are tarot being interpreted towards a sexual question and that the cards do mean other things when drawn in connection with different issues. When I don't offer a reversed interpretation it means that the reversed card doesn't change the meaning that much. In a whole spread surrounding cards will always modify an interpretation and I shall give some examples as we go along.

You'll note that I am starting with the Minor cards. In tarot Major Cards symbolise absolute truths in life that we all live by, while the Minor Cards symbolise how we react to these situations through our own unique personalities. Hence the Minor Cards are far more important when discussing sexual preferences, performance, and the types of people we may encounter.

Let's Start at Basics.

Suit of Batons and sex in tarot

The tarot suit of batons, or wands as some people know them, relate to the element of fire. Fire gives us energy, an ability to perform active tasks and passion. They represent sexual energy.

The Ace of Batons symbolises the erect penis. Therefore the reversed ace of batons symbolises the flaccid penis. This can be sexual dysfunction or erectile problems. The upright ace can also depict your desire for sex or to be sexy, as well as showing that you are the one who initiates sex with your partner.

When discussing their sex life every client is thrilled to see the Ace of Batons, the erect penis. No-one is happy seeing the ace of batons reversed. For men it can mean that there is some sort of erectile dysfunction going on, and one needs to assess whether there is an underlying physical condition or whether it is an emotional issue. For women it can mean that their partner is having problems, or, quite simply; that they aren't getting any.

For either sex it can mean that their libido is low and that they simply don't feel like it.

Let's take an example of how this might be seen in practice. The Ace of Batons reversed next to the Page of Cups reversed often means that there has been, or is, infidelity. Either the one who is being unfaithful no longer wants to have sex with their partner, or the one who was loyal does not wish to have sex with the unfaithful one. In a reading it isn't always necessarily 'the other person' who has been unfaithful; it can equally be the person sitting right across the table from me.

Many women claw back their unfaithful spouse from a mistress, in the belief that it's best for the children, or for financial security, but then don't want to have sex with their partner ever again. It's a lose-lose situation.

Another, often seen, combination is the Ace of Batons reversed next to the four of swords reversed. The four of swords reversed symbolises recovering from feeling unwell, so it's perfectly natural for someone's libido to be low while they're building up their strength.

In a reading the upright ace of batons can be indicative of what turns somebody on. e.g. Next to the Page of Swords they would like dressing up, while next to the Seven Batons they are excited by looks and beauty.

The Two of Batons symbolises domination. Sexually the questioner or their partner might like to use domination as a sexual turn on. This can mean anything from being held down firmly during the sexual act, to employing a dominatrix. It does not, however, include tying up and bondage; that is represented by the Eight of Swords.

When reversed the Two of Batons symbolises release from domination. Domination in sex might be a real turn off for this person, an absolute no, no.

Domination does not always have to be physical and can also be experienced at a mental or emotional level. This is where judging surrounding cards is so important. Does the two of batons sit next to an emotional cups card or a mental swords card? Overall the Two of Batons isn't the friendliest of cards to find in connection to sex. Not many of us like to feel bullied and pressurised when it comes to intimacy, so if this card is shown with regards to a new relationship, it's time to think twice. Does the questioner really want to be 'under the thumb,' and controlled; and only allowed to have sex the way their partner likes it, and only when their partner wants it?

A really negative example would be seeing the Two of Batons placed next to the very strict King of Swords, who likes to get his own way and can be a bully.

A very positive example is seeing the Two of Batons reversed next to the Three of Batons which would indicate a release from old ideas and gaining freedom of sexual expression.

The Three of Batons symbolises fertility, creativity and birth. Oops! We are now getting into the serious side of sex and one or other partner might wish to have sex as a means of conceiving a child. It can also represent artistic forms of sex, such as erotic art... but not necessarily straight pornography. When reversed the Three of Batons suggests that the libido is switched off, (maybe use some of that erotic art to turn it back on) or that sex is denied unless it is to have children.

This is sex at its natural best and the questioner is very, very happy doing their own thing...whatever that might be.

When interpreting tarot we must stay very aware of the position of each card. For example, if we ask the client to take two cards to represent their sex life then we need to watch which card they take first. We must then read the cards in the order they were taken. So, if they take the Two of Batons followed by the Three of Batons this indicates that enjoying sexual domination is part of their nature. If they take the Three of Batons and then the Two of Batons this indicates that a dominant partner spoils their natural ability to go with the flow and inhibits their pleasure.

The Four of Batons symbolises the home, and people with this card rarely like to have sex unless it is in the comfort of bed, or maybe the living room. No outside romps for these folk.

If this card symbolises the questioner's partner, or desired type of partner, it means that they like someone who is homely and domesticated. Not everyone wants to go out clubbing all night, or boozing; some prefer dinner parties or having friends round for summer BBQs, and staying in on rainy days with a DVD. It's warm and cuddly, friendly and laid back.

For example, the Four of Batons next to the King of Cups depicts a man who is a good cook and will use the preparing and serving of fine food as part of his seduction.

The Four of Batons next to the Queen of Cups depicts a woman who enjoys home life and looks to having children as part of her sexual fulfilment.

The Five of Batons symbolises bickering and fluctuating energy. This is a bit of a no go area for any form of positive sex unless the questioner finds nagging a turn on. Also due to its ebb and flow it can mean that the woman is menstruating or suffering from pre-menstrual tension. (p.m.t.) For either sex they may simply be run down, or recovering from a cold.

The other negative side of the Five of Batons is that it represents the chatter-box. There's nothing wrong with talking sexy or lovely-dovey during love-making, or sharing a conversation afterwards, but do you really want to be in bed with someone who talks, and talks, and talks? This type has such a restless mind that right at the point where you're having the most fun they're likely to come out with the most obscure comment about something totally unrelated to the process in hand. Next to the Pope card this issue is exacerbated. Next to the Judgement card they suddenly remember something, or have a great idea, yet feel the need to blurt it out and share it…during sex!

On a more positive note the Five of Batons can symbolise a desire for a change in sexual activity, either more or less, depending on surrounding cards. With the Page of Swords it symbolises a desire to go and find a 'naughty' person for an experimental romp, while next to the Nine of Cups it depicts going out with friends, having some fun and seeing who's new on the scene.

The Six of Batons symbolises a best friend. Very often people have a best, or good friend, of the opposite sex; but generally they like being friends so don't have sex together. Only in the correct context can it mean what I call "occasional company," (some people prefer the phrase fuck-buddy) two good friends who sometimes have sex together; but it is not a "relationship" as such. For long term married couples it indicates that their partner is their best friend as well as lover.

When taking cards for future romance it means that the questioner desires a long term partner who is their best friend, and that in some ways the sex is secondary, and the ability to be friends and share quality time together is the greatest need.

The Seven of Batons symbolises high energy and beauty. This is all about the attraction side of sex. He/she is drop dead gorgeous! Physical attraction is important, and this is the card that gets folk looking at each other and being interested. When reversed the Seven of Batons indicates apathy, and here one simply can't be bothered, or doesn't like the look, or personality, of whoever they have met for a hot date.

I often see this card reversed in what can only be described as tired relationships. The first passions were built on youth and physical appearance, and once those initial attractions have worn away with age the couple discover that they have very little in common that will sustain the relationship.

When the deeper side of this card is in play, and the couple have initially been attracted by the beauty inside the other person, then the Seven of Batons can lead to a highly fulfilled long term relationship. One elderly gentleman had this card to represent his marriage, and once I had explained its meaning he smiled and said, "My wife is the most beautiful human being I have ever met. We have been married over forty years and her light continues to shine through."

The Eight of Batons symbolises sexual excitement and extremes of passion. It's a bit of a wow card! However, reversed it represents lightning speed and sexually that may well prove to be disappointing if the act itself doesn't last very long! A bit "wham-bam thank you ma'am."

In a regular relationship it can mean finding time for a 'quickie,' but overall, because this card is so extreme and intense, its heightened passion is difficult to sustain for any length of time. Steamy is good, but how long can the kettle keep boiling before it runs dry?

I've frequently seen the Eight of Batons next to the Knight of Cups indicating that couples who do not live together, but maintain a long distance relation, keep the excitement and passion going for longer. The Knight of Cups brings in the romantic yearning to see the partner after being absent, so this can also apply when a couple have been separated due to work or family commitments.

The Nine of Batons symbolises strength. This is one for the girls...he is a hunk! He is strong, both physically and emotionally. It shows that a man has staying power and is capable of sustaining an erection and having sex all night long.

When depicting a woman it means that she is fit and healthy and can keep pace in bed.

For both sexes it depicts a healthy lifestyle, enjoying exercise and the great outdoors. Hence these types enjoy having sex out in the woods or fields, or may have met each other at the gym and find that exercise stimulates their sexual appetite.

If the questioner draws this card in response to the question, "How is my relationship?" the indication is that it is strong and can survive all sorts of problems and issues, and will have good staying power.

When the Nine of Batons is reversed it depicts tiredness. Just go to bed and cuddle, one or the other is far too worn out to be sexually active and may even be going down with a cold.

The Ten of Batons symbolises burdens. People who draw this card are so busy they simply don't have time for a sex life! In fact they don't even make time to go out and meet anyone. When reversed the Ten of Batons symbolises taking the first steps towards creating that precious time for love, sex and romance. Pack the kids off for the weekend, turn the phone off, and have some fun.

The upright card can also represent pregnancy, so if you're asking the cards what the outcome of your hot date might be then it's best to make sure you stock up on condoms...and remember to put them in your pocket before you go out. Next to both the Queen of Cups and the Empress the Ten of Batons symbolises high fertility and maternal instincts.

The Ten of Batons can also indicate that someone is over-weight. If the card represents the questioner then they are most likely unhappy with their weight. One very attractive woman drew this card in response to the question, "Why am I having difficulty meeting the right man?" I looked across the table and said, "You look fantastic. Why are you worried about your weight?" She replied, "I used to be slimmer and I don't feel sexy being this size." Consequently we used the reading to explore how she could improve her self-image so that she would feel more confident and attract a partner.

There is, of course, the other side to the story and for one woman I described her future love as a "chubbie-chappie." She groaned with disappointment. Several months later she brought her 'new man' over for a reading. Sure enough, he had a fuller figure. "I never would have crossed the room to speak to him if not for you," she said. "I was always looking for an athletic sort of guy, and never bothered to see what was on the inside." They are now married, and guess what...her husband is one of my greatest fans.

Batons Court Cards - people we might meet.

The King of Batons is ... well ... one of my clients once described him as sex on legs. He is strong, sexy, fun, often sporty, and fit... An all round good guy, and even if you don't fall in love with him he's a great guy to have as a sexual partner. He will ooze confidence and be terrific in any social scene.

When reversed the King of Batons is a bit distracted, less sporty and sometimes great in bed but unable to commit. It all depends on what you are looking for.

The one thing about the King of Batons is that everyone likes him and he is always popular, so even if it's a casual relationship you'll get to meet lots of great people. Just watch out that someone doesn't try and steal him from right under your nose.

In a serious relationship this guy can invoke jealousy, but that is only because he is sociable and will chat to lots of people at a party; which can cause confusion and get you wondering whether or not he truly wants to be with you. After all, he is good looking.

In general he is faithful once committed to a partner.

The Queen of Batons is active, pretty, sexy and creative. She is ripe for pregnancy; so boys be aware! She enjoys sex and is fun to be with. Like the King, the Queen of Batons reversed can also be reluctant to commit.

When the King and Queen of Batons are seen together as a couple they are the happiest couple in the pack. They can work and play together, spark off each other with the same sense of humour, and get along well as friends, not just lovers. This is because they both let each other be who they are, and don't expect them to change or become someone else. Neither partner is 'in charge' of the relationship. They give each other freedom to come and go without jealousy and fear, and create a life together that includes strong friendships with other people. They enjoy going out together, holidaying together; and very often have business interests together. They are by no means identical, and are quite often remarkably different types of people; yet they complement each other. This combination is all about being with your 'other half.'

The Knight of Batons symbolises those all important phone calls, emails and text messages from your lover. When the card is upright they appear, but when reversed the message just isn't getting through, and he or she has probably lost interest in communicating. A new interpretation for this card has sprung up over the past few years…internet dating. Often the entire relationship takes place through distant communication, and when it comes to a face to face meeting the spark simply isn't there.

With the Knight of Batons we also have phone sex, those long tantalising phone calls where we turn each other on; and when it all gets too much jump in the car and drive half the night to fulfil the desire.

The Page of Batons symbolises youngsters, so for older women this is great...a toy boy! For older men it's a young nubile nymph. For some people the idea of having a younger lover just doesn't appeal, but don't fret unless the Page is reversed, then it is childishness and immaturity…which means that he or she needs more experience before becoming a competent lover. Teach them everything you know and they'll keep coming back for more.

The Page of Batons will frequently turn up in a reading when the questioner is fed up with their current lover and looking to start fresh with someone else. The card symbolises new beginnings and feeling young and willing have a go at anything. For women this often occurs once the children have left home and their husband isn't giving them enough attention. This would be seen as the Queen of Cups reversed followed by the Page of Batons.

Because the Page of Batons refers to youthfulness and play it is also associated with sex toys. You are more likely to find this interpretation if you ask the question, 'What kind of toys does my partner enjoy?' Here are a few examples.

Next to the Ace of Batons the woman prefers a straightforward penis shaped dildo. To make that into a vibrator add the Wheel of Fortune.

Page of Batons next to Eight of Swords the toys are geared towards bondage.

Next to The Word card the man enjoys any toy that simulates a vagina.

Next to the Queen of Cups we're looking at breast stimulation such as nipple clamps.

Now the Emotions get Involved

Tarot suit of Cups and sex in tarot.

The suit of Cups relates to the element of water. Water symbolises the emotions due to its bonding quality. This is our ability to love and be loved, to form positive relationships and to be sensitive and caring.

The Ace of Cups symbolises the open heart and in a sexual relationship our ability and desire to include the emotions as well as the body. When reversed the Ace of Cups symbolises coldness and a frosty reception as far as "getting emotionally involved." This may be due to past hurts, or simply wishing to disassociate sex from emotional contact.

If the questioner asks, "Will my new partner love me?" and the Ace of Cups reversed is next to the Eight of Swords, then it will be very difficult, if not impossible for their partner to open up and share their emotions. The Eight of Swords type always find it difficult to talk about their emotions and personal fears, and next to the Ace of Cups reversed it suggests that they have suffered a broken heart in a previous relationship, and are likely to remain closed, or at the very least be extremely cautious. Hard work is required for this combination.

Alternately the Ace of Cups reversed next to the Page of Batons suggests a willingness to be playful and try again, even though a previous partner has broken their heart.

On a physical level the Ace of Cups holds water, so this is the wet vagina, juicy and inviting.

The Two of Cups symbolises being in love. Here sex takes place between two people who are in love, or have just fallen in love. This card is all dewy eyed and smoochy. On first meeting it's that eyes across the room electric connection, the stuff that romantic films are made of.

When the Two of Cups is reversed sex is not likely to be taking place at all. It depicts having fallen out of love, or finding something, or someone, distasteful or unpleasant. The classic phrase is, "I simply don't find my lover attractive anymore." This does not necessarily mean physical repugnance, more that the enquirer has discovered a personality trait that simply turns them off. Not sharing the same sense of humour, not enjoying the same type of film, or not enjoying the same type of food can all turn someone off because they will feel out of sync.; and lacking shared pleasures and emotional enjoyment outside the bedroom. This doesn't mean that we need to enjoy exactly the same things as our partner, but if we fail to click on various points then the romance will die.

Please note that all romantic movies end when the couple get together...on the romantic high point, when the Two of Cups energy is strong and sensual.

Many people say that sharing the same sense of humour is one of the traits that keeps romance alive, and often the Two of Cups next to the Nine of Cups indicates that the couple can laugh and enjoy themselves together with friends.

The Three of Cups is traditionally the marriage card, and these days depicts any committed relationship. However, when sex is on the scene, it could well mean that the questioner is not sleeping with their own partner but someone else's!

If the questioner is enquiring about someone they have just met then the Three of Cups could well mean that the person they are attracted to is already taken. For a more established relationship it will mean that both people are considering it a long term commitment.

Next to the Page of Cups reversed there is definite disloyalty, or infidelity, going on. This poses the question of "what is an affair?"

Is an affair having sex outside of the regular relationship, or is it going for a cup of coffee to talk through a colleague's problems...oh, and they just happen to be the opposite sex? This leaves the regular partner having a relationship with someone who is late home and giving all of that wonderful listening attention to someone else. That, for many, is worse than if they were having sex. Quality time and attention is being given to someone outside the relationship when they should be rushing to get the train home.

The Four of Cups symbolises rejection. Prepare to be snubbed when this card shows itself. Physically it means "don't touch."

Very often the Four of Cups will turn up next to the Page of Cups reversed when one partner suspects that the other is having an affair. They don't want to have physical contact until the matter is resolved. If the card appears next to the Queen of Swords then there is the possibility that the female in the relationship is having difficulties with sex. This can be as simple as period pains or p.m.t.; or something more serious.

One simple every day interpretation for this card is that the individual the Four of Cups represents is turning their back on physical contact due to personal issues outside the relationship. Very often they are afraid that a cuddle will make them burst into tears and show their vulnerability.

When this card is drawn for the direct question, "How will this relationship go?" the answer is, "Looks like you're going to be dumped."

When reversed the Four of Cups symbolises having a hug. Here we see cuddles and curling up on the sofa together, a subtle, emotional intimacy, but no direct sex taking place. It is also tenderness and touching your partner throughout the day, such as holding hands when walking together, which is a delicate form of foreplay that invites greater intimacy later.

Due to the tactile nature of the Four of Cups reversed it also represents massage, and this is something the couple will enjoy as part of their lovemaking.

For men the Four of Cups reversed next to the Ace of Batons near enough guarantees a hand job; and holds promise for a blow job, especially if next to the Queen of Cups who enjoys sucking and kissing and tasting her lover.

The Five of Cups symbolises emotional contact that goes way beyond the physical level. Here the emotions are intense and all encompassing, sometimes to the point of being smothering. This is what one might call being psychically connected. Total connection happens at a soul level during sex when this card is involved.

When upright the Five of Cups refers to intuitively 'knowing' someone, without many words needing to be spoken. The couple will feel 'in tune' with each other and play out this connection by doing things like trying to phone each other at exactly the same moment, meet each other for a drink and both be wearing the same colour sweater; or he'll pull up in the car listening to the same music that she's playing on her stereo. Uncanny?

All of this makes for great sex, because the heart connection is so intense that it can feel like merging and blending with the other person to the point of personal non-existence. You literally become one person. Next to the Nine of Swords, the card of the ultimate orgasm, this is a spectacular combination.

When reversed the Five of Cups takes on a more sinister note. All of that emotional closeness has begun to feel like psychic vampirism. The other person just won't psychically disconnect for a while and give you some personal space. This sets up a bad vibration, and some people have described it as being able to feel the dirt clinging to their partner's soul. If someone is in a regular relationship then the Five of Cups reversed will show itself as that awful feeling when they step through the door and just know that their partner has done something awful that makes them feel guilty; like having sex outside the relationship.

If the Five of Cups reversed is drawn when asking about a new partner then they will most likely be the type who wants to smother and own the questioner, and will have a suspicious mind. When drawn next to the Page of Swords it becomes a sinister combination of somebody untrustworthy wishing to control the questioner by emotional intensity, lies and jealousies. A bit of a bunny boiler!

The Six of Cups symbolises the past, present and future, so during sex the mind dwells on past lovers, or potential future events. Unfortunately with sex this usually comes up as the past...with lots of promises that tomorrow it will be better.

When the Six of Cups is reversed the mind is stuck in the past and therefore unlikely to find any satisfaction while having sex. It can also very much get stuck in what happened 'last time,' so if the question is "Will sex be better with my lover tonight?" quite frankly, if it was bad last night, then tonight will be an action replay.

For people who play out their romance through period costume, such as people who like to dance in rock n' roll gear, or become Saxons at the weekend, then the Six of Cups refers to their clothing and the emotions created by their costume. For some this is a yearning for the past and a positive escape from everyday hustle and bustle. The Page of Swords likes to dress up, so if you draw it next to the Six of Cups and the Nine of Cups, then you'll most likely meet the person of your dreams at a fancy dress party with a historic theme.

Depending on surrounding cards it can depict that a lover from the past returns, especially next to the Knight of Cups, who has a habit of popping in and out of one's life. However, next to the Knight of Cups the Six of Cups can also symbolise someone that we have been in close proximity to in the past, yet never truly met. So if these two cards come up next to each other it's always best to take a third card to clarify the situation.

The Seven of Cups symbolises fantasy. Dream on! Here the sex is all in the mind. Romantic films, books and pornography are all depicted by this card, depending on whether you prefer your dream lover to be dashing Mr Darcy or Miss Hot-and-Horny. When reversed the Seven of Cups depicts dreams coming true - hey! - it looks like you get the man or woman of your dreams.

The Seven of Cups is a delicious card, but when the questioner draws it they must be reminded that although dreaming of sex and romance is terrific fun, that actually doing it is even better. With so many 'invisible' ways to attract a partner these days, such as online dating, online computer games, Facebook and tweeting, someone who draws the Seven of Cups can use a lot of energy imagining what the person at the other end is like, and dreaming up rosy scenarios. Not always, but often, they are disappointed when they get to meet the object of their fantasy in reality. That is a real downer, and I hear the phrases, "He was so sweet in his texts," or, "When it came to face to face conversation she was so boring." These technological romances are mainly depicted when the Seven of Cups is next to a sword card, or the Page of Batons.

We all have fantasies and dreams, it's part of human nature. Mostly we go out and endeavour to fulfil these dreams, and we all have our own unique desires. If anyone reading this is a student of astrology then it's well worth studying the 7th harmonic chart as it depicts the individual's fantasies and what turns them on; everything from their taste in art to how they imagine their life should be.

Interpreting the Seven of Cups is very easy. It literally is fantasy plus the card next to it. So alongside the Queen of Wands the questioner would like an attractive fresh faced partner. Next to the Ace of Swords the priority is to have a truthful, honest partner. Next to the Ten of Batons they prefer someone with a rounder figure.

When reversed the girl/boy of your dreams is in front of you. This is wish fulfilment. Hmmm. Just be careful what you wish for. One client wished and wished for a girlfriend, and when she appeared he was just about to move overseas. "I never wished for right timing, or for the relationship to succeed," he said. "I just wished for her!"

The Eight of Cups symbolises.......oh yipes this is the bored housewife, or fed-up workaholic. Here we find a need to run away from it all. When the questioner pulls this card then they are ripe for some sex outside their regular relationship. When reversed the Eight of Cups depicts an inability to fly loose and let rip even though they feel like it.... shear frustration.

When the questioner draws the Eight of Cups next to the Knight of Cups they are being invited to lead a much more exciting life by an old flame, or someone with foreign connections; or to go on journeys to find new love. I have often seen this combination when the questioner is in an established relationship but their partner does not want to go out, or does not enjoy the same activities. They therefore take off on their own, or are easily persuaded away by someone who has more enthusiasm for life.

The reversed Eight of Cups symbolises someone who is afraid to bring change into their life and meet the world head on. They would truly like to be more daring and tend to come up with a thousand excuses as to why they can't. Sex is often about going to places we have never been before, sexually, emotionally and intellectually, but with the reversed Eight of Cups fear of the unknown gets in the way and makes one stick to 'safe' and consequently stale.

Upright the Eight of Cups is an ability to let go, release and have an orgasm. Reversed the Eight of Cups individual is too afraid to let go and have an orgasm, through fear of the emotional connection letting go might bring.

The Nine of Cups symbolises friends and parties. A convivial atmosphere, mates, a few drinks... not great for sex, but an enjoyable social scene in which to attract someone. If you choose this card it's letting you know that this is the right time to go out and have some fun. It might also imply that some group sex would do you good too!

For couples in committed relationships it's the need for social stimulation. Being intimate is great, but it needs to be balanced with other activities otherwise staying in and having sex every night can become as dull as having no sex at all.

The Nine of Cups also refers to moderate drinking, just a glass or two of wine or a beer; and for any couple this can help relaxation and sexual desire, especially after a hard day's work.

The Ten of Cups symbolises contentment. Here one is content to have some gentle sex, loving emotions, kind words and big hugs. Very soothing, very satisfying.

I often see this card in the readings of people who have been together for a very long time, are truly compatible, and enjoy a mutually satisfying sex life. If you turn the card when asking about future relationships it suggests that you too can find someone who is a perfect match.

Cups Court Cards - people we might meet.

The King of Cups is an absolute sweetie. Often known as the perfect father this guy is loving and kind, but also keen to settle down and start looking after you and the kids. He's not the kind of guy you mess with on a one night stand because he is just far too sensitive and would easily get hurt. When he does the love-sex thing he does it for real, and for keeps. When the King of Cups is reversed he is likely to be a "Mummy's boy" and very emotionally needy. At first it might feel great because this guy will phone and will want to see you...he will need you, apparently desire you; but after a while you'll start to feel smothered and realise that love and sex are all about his wants and his needs, and yours can go a begging.

On a positive note he's very sensuous and likes stroking and touching. In many ways he's shy and hates the idea of rejection, and worries that his advances may not be good enough; so just make sure he gets round to the penetration or he'll spend all evening getting you excited about something that might not happen. He needs reassurance and a little encouragement, so praise his efforts.

If you're a foody then this is the guy for you because he loves cooking and sharing food, so foreplay can take place through the sensuality of the mouth, the tongue and kisses. But make sure he gets round to the main course and dessert.

The Queen of Cups is genuinely loving and kind. She'll make you dinner, listen to your problems; then slowly give you a long soothing massage before taking you to bed. Yum- yum. When reversed the Queen of Cups can be very stand-offish as far as sex is concerned. She wants everything to be "just right" and will appear highly-strung and over sensitive. If you're not careful you'll work hard and then blow it at the last minute, sending her into a mood which it can take until breakfast to shift.

Sex for this woman has to start with the emotions and work down. Be kind, be gentle, and she'll make you feel wonderful.

In a man's reading, next to the Seven of Batons, (visual stimulation) it means that the man likes breasts and this is what will turn him on the most.

The Knight of Cups likes to be free to come and go at will. He or she is enigmatic and exciting, but not always able to hang around for long. This is the weekend lover or long distance romance. Sometimes they are so busy being elsewhere that they don't turn up at all...or turn up late! As in, so late that you've missed the party, dinner or other exciting event, and you end up with the impression that you've been kept hanging around while they have fun and that you're only good for sex. When the Knight of Cups is reversed... Well they just don't show up at all, and sometimes don't even bother to phone and apologise.

On a more positive note the Knight of Cups also depicts foreign lovers and romance while overseas. It can also symbolise an old flame returning to your life, or someone you have vaguely met in the past but never spoken to. e.g. you'll discover that you used to live three doors away but never noticed them.

The Knight of Cups is an exciting and adventurous card and also shows when you're ready to explore new horizons and different lovers. It's the card of 'finding what turns you on," so don't be afraid to experiment. Next to the World card the Knight of Cups is ready to get out into the world, maybe even 'come out' if gay; so it's time to show the world who you really are.

The Page of Cups is loyal and faithful. Sometimes this Page can be a little bit of a push-over because they are so keen to please, but hey, that isn't always such a bad thing when sex is involved. When reversed the Page of Cups is unfaithful and disloyal. I have seen this so often when someone in a long term relationship has had an affair, and what's worse is that they are likely to bitch about it, accusing their partner of this and that as a way of making excuses for their own behaviour. "They were too needy," "They wanted so much from me," are typical reversed Page of Cups complaints.

This loyal Page of Cups is a servant and gives good service, so it may also represent a prostitute who is being paid for a sexual service. However, it also represents nurses and can show that someone likes dressing up as a nurse as a turn on. Ooh Matron!

With the next two suits of Coins and Swords we move away from the sensual, emotional world of the physical act and into the complexities of daily life, mind games and money, all of which have the ability to influence our joy of sex or ability to perform.

Sexual Values

Tarot suit of Coins and sex in tarot

The suit of Coins, or pentacles as some people like to call them, relate to earth. This suit is all about how we survive in the physical world, wisdom and wealth; money and knowledge; and whether or not we possess a core sense of security.

The Ace of Coins symbolises ownership, the legal side of relationship, that all meaning piece of paper. The Cups may well bond us together, but this is the document that says, 'you are mine,' the marriage certificate. For some this is an important stage of personal release to their partner, an assurance of fidelity; while to others it's the proverbial mill-stone around their neck. Oh gosh, the mill-stone is round too, like the coin. The bottom line is that money changes hands in exchange for sex, but don't get me wrong, we're not just talking prostitution, this happens all of the time in marriage as well as out on the streets. The husband buys the wife a new car…in the hope of receiving sex. The young man buys his new girlfriend a meal…in the hope of receiving sex. You get the picture.

The Two of Coins symbolises vacillation, a dithering this way and that. Do we want sex tonight or not? Do we want to have that affair or not? Here it's all related to the consequences of the act, as in, what will be the result of having sex with this individual? If you are married, will having great sex with you persuade them to leave their partner, or will you be left a fool?

This card can also depict uncertainty regarding sexual orientation. Straight or gay, straight or bi-sexual, the questioner is uncertain, and unwilling to step forwards into new experiences for fear of fallout and loss of face in the world.

It can also mean dithering in the bedroom, quite simply, should we do this or that? For goodness sake, get on with it!

The Three of Coins symbolises being the one in the driving seat of a relationship. Unfortunately if one person is the boss then it is never an equal partnership. Of course, it can also mean sleeping with your boss, which is often a recipe for disaster.

When reversed the card depicts being a people pleaser, a yes person, and this creates two forms of complication. Firstly the individual may fall into the trap of performing sexual acts they, personally, are unhappy with, in order to please their partner. Secondly, when they fail to please, or decide not to please any more, the partner will reject or criticise them. Back in your box, stay subservient, or lose. But hey, what is there to lose if it isn't any fun?

The Three of Coins upright is also about teaching and learning. You may be the teacher or the student. It will especially have this interpretation when next to one of the Page cards, showing that one person is younger than the other, and is prepared to learn a few tricks from their more experienced partner. However, the reversed card will still show that your partner is teaching you what they want you to know in order to please them, and not you.

The Four of Coins symbolises security. Dull, boring, keep doing the same old stuff in bed because we know it works and gets results. It isn't exciting, but it can be fulfilling. Money is behind this card too, showing that as long as the individual has enough money in the bank and a nice home then they can perform. Take that away and they won't be able to get their act together.

For both men and women it can mean that they do not wish to have sex with someone unless they appear to be prosperous.

The Five of Coins depicts help along the way. Generally I have seen this card in situations where someone needs a friend in order to go out and pull; someone to give them support to get out and meet people. When reversed there is no-one to go out with…in all senses of the term. On many occasions I have seen this card depict relationships in which the two people have 'rescued and saved' each other after difficult times. i.e. they have both just finished unhappy marriages. Sometimes these new relationships last, but more often than not the couple drift apart once they are healed from the pain.

For the sex act itself it can mean that some practical support is required. Most often in the form of Viagra or additional lubrication.

The Six of Coins symbolises balance of payments and favours. When upright it shows that the amount of effort you put into the relationship, and the sexual side of it, is equally balanced by your partner. When reversed it shows that you are putting in more effort than your partner, and therefore feeling unrewarded. The reversed cards talks of being 'ripped off,' someone has taken advantage, and in the bedroom this becomes highly unsatisfactory. The phrase I most often hear is, "I feel used." The partner is getting all of the sexual gratification, while you are not.

If we go back to the young man I mentioned in the Ace of Coins who buys his new girlfriend dinner in the hope of being rewarded with sex, when she refuses the Six of Coins reversed will turn up. All of his hard earned cash has been wasted, because he wasn't rewarded for his efforts.

The Six of Coins reversed will also show up if your partner doesn't bother to say thank you for sex, or gets up and leaves the room without a word. It may sound crazy to thank your partner for sex, but the words, 'That was great,' will do. It's not about praise; it's about gratitude for the shared intimacy.

Rocking backwards and forwards during sex, and also swinging (as in, being on a swing-not wife swapping) are shown with the upright card.

The reversed Six of Coins has to come with a warning if this card is drawn to ask about a first date. Beware, it can mean that someone is having sex with you because they want to steal your possessions. It's usually pre-meditated, so they'll get into your bed and have sex with the deliberate intention of taking something from your home before they leave; usually small items such as money from your wallet, your favourite C.D. or the toothpaste.

Next to the Four of Batons: theft from your home.

Next to the Nine of Coins: theft from hotel you go to have sex in.

Next to Page of Swords: theft from your clothing i.e. jacket or handbag.

The Seven of Coins symbolises work. Ok, so all relationships are work and need to be worked on. All sex has to be learnt. Sure, it comes naturally, but without some knowledge we're floundering around in the dark; acting on lust, impulse and nature. So, we need to learn technique, maybe read some books, watch some "how to" T.V. programmes; and discover what our partner does and doesn't enjoy. Everyone you have sex with is different, so learn what they like' and don't come out with the old phrase, "But my last girlfriend/boyfriend really liked me doing that." You'll mostly hear that phrase when the Seven of Coins is reversed next to the Six of Cups reversed.

When reversed the card depicts work that we do but don't feel much like doing….and, quite frankly, if we're doing that with sex…then what are we doing there in the first place? If he wants a hand job and you find it goes on and on forever, stop! If she likes three hours of foreplay by which time you're ready to fall asleep, stop! If this was the day job then work is going nowhere, and likewise with sex; you may never get your partner to an orgasm, regardless of how much effort you put in.

The Eight of Coins symbolises a good reputation. Sounds like Casanova, but wait, best put the brakes on here. I saw this card come up for one woman's new boyfriend. Oh sure, he had an excellent reputation as a lover…because he'd been with so many women before her! Sure, sure, it can also depict 'a nice person', but when reversed it truly is the card of the bad reputation and the bad boy/bad girl who is best avoided, unless you enjoy being taken for a ride. Many people say, 'I can change him/her,' but often the eight of coins reversed type has jumped into bed with someone else before the month is out.

With the Eight of Coins we also show off our goods. So for a woman it's wearing a low cut top to show off her breasts and for a man it's showing off, well, whichever part he thinks is best. It's all about putting what's on offer in the shop window...and wrapping it nicely.

The Nine of Coins symbolises long term security. For some the only way to have great sex is in the knowledge of what tomorrow might bring. To know that in the morning your lover will still be in bed beside you, to be assured that he/she will return home from work to you, and only you. When reversed the card depicts emotional insecurity and abandonment issues. Very often people drawing this card in connection with their relationships and sex life were abandoned when young, or bullied and made to feel insecure. They fret about not being good enough, and often appear to be possessive, when in fact they are frightened and worried about being dumped. Treat them with care because they are genuinely sensitive and need that reassuring phone call to say you'll be home late. In bed never compare this individual to your last lover…because the relationship will never be the same again, they will always feel second best.

The Ten of Coins symbolises family and morals. If your Dad told you that masturbation would make it drop off or shrivel up then you'll replay all of that early programming in the bedroom. If the dos and don'ts were geared towards negative, then sex can become a minefield of unconscious worry and concern over crossing invisible boundaries.

Conversely if the family of upbringing spoke of sex as loving and caring then you'll be the one ensuring your partner is treated with respect and tenderness.

The Ten of Coins also symbolises that the questioner has a very strong family background so anyone involved with this individual must expect to spend a lot of time popping round to Mum or Dad's and dutifully attending every family function. They also strongly believe in tradition and would expect to have children to extend the family line.

Often the family's religious ethics and morals come into play, so a Catholic might well refuse to wear a condom because sex is for having babies.

Coins Court Cards - people we might meet.

The King of Coins is a business man, and will tend to treat sex with exactly the same attitude. He sees sex as an exchange of goods, so will expect to be rewarded for taking you out for that expensive meal, or paying the mortgage. If you like to be treated well then this is the guy for you. He will buy tasteful gifts to show gratitude, pay for expensive holidays, but never be around much as he works so hard. In bed he can be adventurous (after all it's his clever thinking that makes all of that money), but will hate making love if he has money worries.

Believe it or not he is very likely to have an affair. Why? Because he is busy working away from home, so has available time, and a good excuse to be out late; and often classes the wife and children as a long term investment. If you're his mistress you'll be treated wonderfully…but he'll never leave his wife. I've heard about this guy from both sides of the story, from the wife who's discovered her husband's having an affair, and from the kept mistress. In at least half of the situations the King Of Coins had purchased a flat either for the mistress, or as a second home (which his wife knew nothing about) so that he had comfort in which to conduct his affair.

The King of Coins reversed is mean and will only spend money if he will be the sole beneficiary. Even in marriage he prefers the house to be in his name alone. In divorce he's cruel and hides money away so that he gives his wife and children as little as legally possible. During sex he's demanding, will make out that his efforts are for you, but in truth it's all about what turns him on. If he's getting on a bit and takes ages and ages to climax you won't be given the option of stopping and trying again tomorrow, regardless of how sore you're getting. He wants the full meal and he will get it. If he doesn't then money or treats will be slyly removed.

The Queen of Coins is a business woman, and often works in accounts. To her sex is all about the odds of gaining long term security, and she aims for committed relationships. In bed she will please her partner, but never cross her own acceptable boundaries. I have seen this card come up for women who marry older men, in their final years of life, as an agreeable trade off - companionship, sex, and caring; in exchange for inheritance.

If you are female and friendly with the Queen of Coins beware as she is the matchmaker, someone who is always looking out for your best interests and will set you up with wealthy suitors. She will constantly veer you away from that heady emotion called true love, and that younger man you have a fixation on. After all, they do not spell out commitment and security.

If you tumble into bed with this woman and the next morning she discovers that you're poor, don't expect a repeat performance.

Like the King reversed the Queen of Coins reversed can also be very selfish and mean. She's someone you admire for her drive and tenacity, but rarely the subject or erotic dreams and fantasies; unless you're into the dominatrix type who says, 'Go and buy me that expensive bracelet, right now.'

The Knight of Coins isn't on the lookout for sex, or romance, and is far more concerned with the overall game plan that they have drawn out for their life. If that includes marriage then they will hit their chosen age for 'settling down' and expect to instantly come up with the right person. Dream on! Frustrated and thwarted they arrive on my doorstep bewildered as to why their well thought out plan isn't working in practice. If you're unlucky enough to meet them when they're still in the working, or playing stage of their master plan, then they will simply say, 'I'm not intending to settle down until I'm blah age,' and gallop away, oblivious of what they are missing.

When reversed the knight of coins has lost the plot and doesn't have plans, or the things they were headed for in life no longer hold meaning. They may well say, 'I don't know where I'm at right now,' and please trust that they mean it, because once they decide on a new route you may well find that you don't fit into the equation; or you're expected to uproot your entire life to follow their dream.

During the sexual act itself the Knight of Coins will always have a plan, and the quality of sex all depends on precisely what their master plan is. If their plan is for their sexual gratification alone then you'll be left unsatisfied and frustrated, but if it's to give you the best orgasm ever then you're in luck. The trouble is you won't know what their plan is until you're half way through and have sussed the plot.

If the Knight of Coins has decided to have sex doggy-style all night, then that is what they want. If you desire more intimacy and the missionary position half way through; it will put them off. You'll swap position, they'll be discontent; you'll go back to the first position, and then they'll moan that it doesn't feel the same anymore.

The Page of Coins is the inveterate gambler, someone who is keen to take risks and see which way the coin will land. Also a renowned ditherer, they rarely decide on an act quickly and efficiently. As far as sex goes this makes them a weird mixture of impulsive and non-active. The gambler side will jump into bed with the most unlikely of partner, willing to take a risk on where it might lead, while the ditherer side will hum and hah while the boy/girl of their dreams is swept away by Perfect Charming. Putting the two sides together they can appear terribly contradictory, leaping into bed and sex, and then spending the following few hours debating whether or not it was a mistake, and should it have happened in the first place?

During sex they will come up with creative ideas and then, half way through, suddenly try something different just as you were getting off on it. They will also fiddle and faff, wondering if the pillows, lighting, and music should be softer, dimmer or quieter…while you quickly go off the boil.

The reversed Page of Coins is pretty much a non-starter. They don't want to take a gamble, are far too worried about making a mistake, and more often than not never get round to the business in hand. If you share a bed with the page of Coins reversed and actually sleep then you'll have a disturbed night because they'll toss and turn and be the most fidgety person you've ever been with. Phew, tiring.

Mind Games & Intellectual Pursuits

Tarot suit of Swords and sex in tarot

The suit of Swords relate to air. This suit is all about the mind and those twisting turning complexities of the human thought process. Not always a good bed fellow when ideas, both old and new, get in the way of spontaneous creativity.

The Swords rule knives, needles and many other shiny pointy Items, hence body piercings are depicted through this suit.

The Ace of Swords symbolises truth, honesty and integrity. So, they're honest, which is a bonus; but they can also want things done their way, because that is how they understand sex. They can also be terribly blunt when communicating emotions. "Did you just fake that orgasm?" you ask. "Yes, of course, you were useless," they will reply, and follow through with, "Well, you asked, and I was honest," even though it cuts you to the core.

The reversed Ace is the exact opposite offering fibs, lies and a damn good cover up. This is great if you want to believe their little fib that you were a terrific lover, but if you're asking whether they're in a relationship before bedding them and the reversed ace of swords pops up…buyer beware!

The Two of Swords symbolises keeping the peace, tension and unspoken upsets. Most likely you're already in a relationship, of some kind, with this man or woman before having sex with them, because here the entire act can be spoilt by smouldering discontent; because you didn't sit down and discuss those pressing issues before taking them to bed. Oops! If you're not already in relationship and this card comes up then a prickly tension will fill the atmosphere, most likely once you've given that heady romp your all, and he/she clambers out of bed exuding bad vibes. But why? What did you do? You'll never know, because the two of swords will always prefer to create stress than be the one to cast the first blow and become the 'bad guy.' They'd much rather you do that by prodding and poking and making a scene.

When reversed you'll get half way through and they won't be able to go any further until 'it' is sorted out. Oh boy, best get your trousers back on and make a cup of tea. While you're in the kitchen don't forget the can opener to let out all of those worms, because prising stuff out is going to be painful and take forever.

There's also an element of 'giving in' with the Two of Swords. Maybe you didn't enjoy going down on your lover last time, and now they've just said how much fun it was and would love some more. So you oblige, just to keep the peace, even though you find it distasteful.

The Three of Swords symbolises, anger, revenge, jealousy and hatred. Ok, so some people do get their jollies by being angry and then enjoy great sex while making up; but overall this card is not conducive to sex, so if you've lit the blue touch paper you'd best stand well back. No, don't put the kettle on, they'll yell even louder if you dare try and walk away.

When this card means revenge it can seriously make you question why they are bedding you in the first place. Because you broke their heart, and they're showing that they can 'still have you,' before dumping you? Because they're sleeping with you to get at your husband/wife, partner, or past lover? There is usually history attached to the situation when the three of swords symbolises revenge; so make sure you know who you're jumping into bed with if this card shows its ugly face.

Jealousy is a demon. Are you being treated badly because they don't believe that the man or woman you were seen having coffee with was only a friend? Suspicion makes this lover's blood curdle and they simply don't trust you. Only you know whether their suspicions hold any truth. If they don't then this individual has most likely been treated badly in the past...or they're jealous by nature and prone to such outbursts, with the real possibility of ending up separating you from friends of the opposite sex. (or same sex if you're gay)

Hatred is an unwelcome bed fellow. Is it you they hate, their colleague at work, or themselves?

When reversed all of the anger, revenge, jealousy and hatred is suppressed, creating so much tension that the recipient simply won't be able to work out what's going on. Why isn't the sex as good as it used to be? What gripe are they holding onto like a baby's comforter? Best force the issue and get it out into the open, even if it does mean make or break.

The Four of Swords symbolises places of retreat and healing. Yippee we've arrived at the bedroom! Plain and simple, somewhere you can slip away to, out of sight from the world and prying eyes, so that you can be intimate together. For some it's the fields, the car park, or a ruined building, wherever opportunity offers an element of privacy. Of course, if you're having a fling with your boss, it could be the stationary cupboard.

The reversed Four of Swords is all about sexual healing. Many of us get hurt, physically, mentally or emotionally in our genitals, and need to be healed so that we can experience a fulfilling sexual life again, or even for the first time. Women can be torn or damaged during childbirth and require tenderness and understanding so that they can have intercourse again, even once the physical body has healed. I saw this so clearly for one couple when I was reading for the husband at a weekend retreat. Fortunately he was honest and open and admitted that no sex had taken place since the birth of their third child. He had assumed that his wife had just 'gone off it,' and was being a bit hormonal, even though the child was over a year old. When I explained about the need for healing in their intimate life, he agreed to get into the Cups side of sex and start with stroking and cuddling; something he had avoided doing. The very next day I saw the couple together and they both greeted me with smiles and hugs and kisses. The wife was just so happy. "I only needed a little encouragement," she said, and her husband grinned like a Cheshire cat.

Without the Tarot and the understanding that a sexual healing needed to take place they might have remained apart sexually for many more months.

For others it is not so simple. For some the sexual damage goes right back to childhood, and I have seen this for men who have been circumcised as a baby; who not only experience a lack of sensitivity, but also burning resentment at being defiled. For both sexes I have seen cases of childhood sexual abuse that still require healing, even though they are now in long term sexually active relationships. In these deep rooted cases professional help is required, as well as a loving partner.

When the Four of Swords reversed is next to the Five of Cups the combination refers to tantric sex and the healing power of the couple experiencing sex at a higher spiritual/emotional level.

The Five of Swords symbolises persuasion and mental manipulation. With this card comes a feeling of pressure; that you're being mentally forced into a situation that you're not entirely happy with, and would probably prefer not to continue. There isn't any physical force involved here, no rape or violence, but a horrid sense that if you don't comply that something might happen, even if it's only anger. "Have another drink," they say, knowing that you'll be too drunk to know what you're doing. "I bought you dinner," they say, turning on the guilt. "It's okay, I don't have any sexual diseases," he says, refusing to wear a condom. "Don't bother with a condom, I'm on the pill," she says, but doesn't mean it, or mention how many other guys she's said that to. Are these starting to make you feel uncomfortable?

This card can, of course, take place during sex itself, with your lover persuading you to become involved in their sexual preferences. "I've always wanted to tie someone up and have sex, wouldn't you love that?" No, you probably wouldn't. It hasn't been discussed beforehand and now you're in the bedroom and he's got some fluffy pink handcuffs that he's waving in your direction. There's nothing wrong with a bit of bondage if that is what you both would like and enjoy, but this card takes place at the last minute, when there isn't time to back out without creating a scene. It's manipulation, not discussion.

The Five of Swords also represents religious beliefs and sometimes what is acceptable in the eyes of one man's god is not permitted by another's. Your religious proclivities may not deny you rolling around in the hay with each other, but it may flag up taboos that are insurmountable and create not only inner turmoil but also disgust and abhorrence.

The Six of Swords symbolises analysis and over thinking. Some folk like it quick and easy, but in contrast the over concerned Six of Swords type wants it to be perfect, so they plan it all out like a military campaign. What if this, or that, goes wrong? The bed must be perfect and the lighting must be perfect, and then they allocate enough time for kissing and foreplay and... so don't you dare rush them by wanting it faster or slower. I always think of this card as the mechanic, because in bed it's all a bit mechanical.

Oh, and then there's the cleanliness side of the Six of Swords. "Did you wash your penis?" No? "Well you can use the bathroom now, if you like." And just as you got an erection, what a turn off. Don't panic, men are cleanliness freaks too, and all the sweet perfumes in the world won't convince them that you'll do as you are. Yep, you know where the bathroom is.

Some cleanliness freaks will cleverly disguise their fastidiousness as foreplay, that's when you see the Six of Swords next to the Four of Cups reversed and they'll run a long hot bath for you both, or suggest you have fun together under the shower.

The Six of Swords reversed is over analytical and you'll finish sex only to plough into a blow by blow account of what has just occurred, how it can be improved upon, and which bits could be left out next time. This is sexual dissection, and just when you felt chilled out and ready to doze off.

Because they're highly intellectual the Six of Swords type will also be a wealth of facts and figures, which they love sharing during sex. The moment of orgasm is upon you and they say, "Did you know they used to make condoms out of sheep's gut?" At a time like that...who cares!

The Seven of Swords is all about the go between. The most negative side of this card is when two people have been really angry and upset with each other, so much so that they simply can't speak to the other person. Time passes and the situation rots and eventually has to be cleared up so that everyone can return to having some sex. Cue the mediator who will liaise between one side and the other. Not sexy at all. The more pleasant side is when we ask a friend to speak to the object of our desire and arrange an introduction. "Hey, see that drop dead gorgeous guy, go and ask if he's got a girlfriend." And if he hasn't I can go and chat him up. Again, no sex, but at least there's hope.

One particularly nasty combination of cards is the Three of Swords next to the Seven of Swords. This is where someone is playing out sexual revenge through a third person, and often the middle man or woman is an innocent pawn in someone else's evil plan. I have seen this where a guy sleeps with a girl and is rude and never speaks to her again, because the girl's ex has said, "She's easy," or "She's a hard-nosed bitch," but in truth is neither and is genuinely looking for love and companionship. The girl ends up extremely upset, and doesn't even know why the guy was so nasty to her, until, maybe months or years later, she discovers that her ex had a word in his ear.

If you see this combination of cards for a future relationship, don't even go there. Once you split up he, or she, will want revenge, and maybe even public humiliation.

The Eight of Swords symbolises inner torture. Believe it or not sex can, and does, occur when this card is in play, but the non eight of swords partner feels that the other person is 'not connected' and holding back their emotions. I have had hundreds of people bring this issue to my table, and they say that their partner is distant and not 'letting them in.' For positive, delightful sex, to take place, two people need to trust and permit access to parts of their being that no other person shares. The physical body is merely the outer casing, the vehicle by which pleasure is received, but the mind is the stimulus, the gateway to the soul.

The Eight of Swords type has experienced pain and heartache in the past, very often from an early age, and been told to shut up and keep quiet about their problems. Hence they daren't share inner thoughts for fear of ridicule. When the Eight of Swords is reversed it is the first tentative steps towards voicing their concerns, so let them speak and connect via the mind before involving the body. They are sensitive, and caring, and well worth the trouble.

On a purely physical level the Eight of Swords symbolises vaginal dryness. Even though the individual gets turned on the juices simply refuse to flow. Best option, reach for the lubrication.

Next to The World card reversed the Eight of Swords can represent vaginismus, where the muscles of the vagina tighten involuntarily when vaginal penetration is attempted. This is mostly due to psychological factors, but can include medical issues. Professional help is required.

For both men and women there is dryness in the lower regions and the other sexual problem that occurs is constipation. Yes, sex when really constipated is no fun at all, and a lot of abdominal discomfort can occur. Best option, prune juice; get those bowels moving.

Another sexual side of things for women with the Eight of Swords is lack of blood flow during menstruation. These days some women take a contraceptive pill that stops the periods altogether. Now that's great, because it means she's available for sex 24/7, however, the real down-side which, trust me, I have seen in many readings, is a lack of sexual libido. With this condition it's best to consult your G.P. about an alternative contraceptive pill, or a completely different form of contraception.

The Eight of Swords can also depict people who enjoy bondage and tying up as part of their love making. Very often when next to the Page of Swords or the Two of Batons, although with the Two of Batons it is not so likely to be a fun experience, because domination is included, but if that is what turns you on, then that's fine too.

The Nine of Swords symbolises mental anguish and the mind is giving way. Sounds dreadful for sex, but in fact it's the complete opposite. This is death, the end of separation. This is the ultimate orgasm!

Most human beings believe that they are the mind, their thoughts and ideas. In order to connect with another human being we must let go of ourselves and surrender everything. When we permit this to happen we merge and blend and become one with our lover, and die as an individual. In French it is called Le Petite Mort, The Little Death, that moment of absolute bliss where we are not even aware that we are someone other than our lover.

For the Nine of Swords there are other, more brutal and terrifying interpretations, where sex is concerned. To see this in anyone's reading is rare, and in all my years as a reader have only witnessed it in a few readings, mainly for women whose husbands or lovers were seriously mentally disturbed and prone to violent outbursts. Very often drink or drug fuelled madness is brought to the bedroom, and rather than pleasure the recipient is terrified and ends up believing that they must be the one who is insane.

Couple the Nine of Swords with the Eight of Swords and we start to see some very unsavoury scenarios. Bondage with violence. Is that fun, or is that rape? Is he holding you down and forcing himself upon you, or is he so uptight and drunk that he's being brutal?

The Ten of Swords symbolises days of sadness and depression. This card cuts both ways and depends highly on the type of individual who draws it. Some people desire sex when they are depressed as a way of adding meaning to their life, while others hide in their cave and daren't go there. For a sexual interpretation of the ten of swords always carefully assess the cards surrounding it.

Swords Court Cards - people we might meet.

The King of Swords is prone to be ruthless in his pursuit of precisely what he desires. He isn't unkind, but he is to be obeyed. His autocratic manner is best suited to work, and this card is more likely to represent someone's career status than their sexual attitudes. If you do manage to prise him away from his busy work schedule be prepared to encounter someone who is cool and austere, likely to make love with the lights off and not prone to smoochy pillow talk. Although somewhat emotionless in his approach he is conscientious, the type who needs to see a result and will expect to see you climax first...because he hates failure. Unfortunately your orgasm will be administered via fingers and tongue, penetration saved for his pleasure, by which time you've probably shut down and fancy some kip.

The King of Swords reversed is generally far too uptight to consider sex. Sometimes there are health issues in the abdomen and genital area which have made them switch off their sex life. Constipation, urinary infections and erectile dysfunction can all be culprits. However, I have also seen the King of Swords reversed when the man is healed of his embarrassing condition, yet the mind hangs on to what did happen, and so his entire body finds it impossible to relax and enjoy sex again.

The Queen of Swords is very often not getting it for one reason or another. On the mental and emotional side she is feeling hurt, upset or just plain angry with you; so much so that she's climbed into her shell and doesn't want physical contact. Very often she is alone or lonely, even when in a relationship. Sometimes the partner has cheated on her, and although she's accepted him back the idea of letting him touch her after he's been having rumpy-pumpy with some nubile nymph from the office is more than she can take. So why have him back in the first place?

On a physical level she experiences sex as uncomfortable, painful or distasteful. Very often there is a real issue going on down below, or in the uterus, so if this unfortunate lady is your partner or wife, I would strongly recommend some tenderness, open discussion and a prompt visit to your G.P. I have seen this card represent everything from minor cases of thrush to more serious ovarian cancer. So if you draw this card and sex is painful, get it checked out.

The Knight of Swords is a man, or woman, on a mission, determined to win the love of their life, or to get laid for the night. (no pun intended) The cards that follow the Knight of Swords indicate what he's aiming for, so study them closely, and you'll discover if it's you he's after.

When reversed this card represents a battle lost, and weariness in the pursuit of one's goal. Is it just too difficult to make him or her reach a climax? Are you convinced that you're incompatible in the sack? Usually the knight of swords will resume his mission after rest, reflection and encouragement.

The Page of Swords is the most complex and intriguing card in the pack. He has so many facets to his personality, and many of them geared towards sex, that you'll never truly know where you stand with him. By the way, he can depict a man or a woman; and most things in between.

With the Page of Swords you never get what you expect. What you see is definitely not what you get.

He likes dressing up and is a true peacock, so for boys and girls of all ages this card is about putting on your glad rags and going out on the pull. He, or she, also likes dressing up in their partner's clothes, and when taken a stage further the Page of Swords represents cross dressers and transvestites.

Due to his ability to appear to be something he is not the Page of Swords can be homosexual, lesbian or bi. Unless we're down in Brighton or a gay bar we assume that a guy is a guy and a girl is a girl, and that we are chatting up a person of the opposite sex, who might fancy us. Gay people don't go around with labels, so we simply don't know, until they tell us, or introduce us to their partner.

Completely separate from any sexual preferences the Page of Swords is a mental gymnast and loves playing mind games. He can be very sweet one moment and scathingly cruel the next. When taken to extremes this type enhances their personality with drink or drugs, making themselves more outrageous, or brighter and quicker when fuelled by stimulants. Very often his addiction is the mood swinger, one drink too many sending Mr Nice Guy into a snarling menace. (this goes for girls as well)

It's also the card that represents teenagers, who love to experiment with all of these things.

As a lover the Page of Swords can be exciting, and unpredictable, but more often than not their unpredictability makes them predictable. You come to expect them to let you down, or to turn up drunk, or to have spent their money on clothes. In bed they're thrilling, until their mood suddenly changes and their loving words hold a sinister tone. Are they playing a mind game or do they really mean to upset you? You'll never know, and mostly they won't either.

The Major Cards and Sex

In Tarot the Major Cards symbolise absolute truths in life that we all live by. They are archetypes. The Minor Cards show how we, as unique individuals, react to these. This is why the minor suits have more impact on us sexually; because they are personal. This does not mean that the Major Cards never show their face in relation to a client's sexual activities, but more often they indicate a 'type' of person, or that the client is working through some major issue and unconsciously sex, and their sexuality, is playing a vital role.

The Major Cards are illustrated with male and female figures, and for the sake of simplicity I shall refer to them by the gender depicted on the card, but do remember that any Major Card can symbolise either sex.

No 0 The Fool symbolises the free spirit and he is just as likely to easily walk away from an unsatisfactory relationship as to plunge head first into a new one. Thought doesn't come into it where the Fool is concerned, he just knows when something is right or wrong.

The word taboo doesn't fit well in his vocabulary and where sex is concerned if he feels like trying something different he'll suggest it, or, if single, go out and find it. Freedom is his catch phrase, so he lives and let's live, not worrying about what others are up to, as long as everyone is happy with their own sexuality. The Fool will never intentionally hurt anyone, but if he needs 'some space' he pretty well needs it now, and hates feeling trapped.

When reversed the Fool does feel trapped, stifled and like a caged tiger. Most often I've seen this when one half of a married couple wishes to try something different in bed, and their partner says 'no go'. I saw this for one guy who admitted that he'd given up bondage once he'd married, thinking he could live without it, but as the years rolled on he found that sex without his own particular turn on was less and less satisfactory. His wife just didn't want to tie him up. Eventually the Fool broke free and they divorced, ending up best friends.

For others I've seen it as the simple fact that they couldn't have sex when they wanted it. If your partner says 'not tonight honey,' what do you do?

No 1 The Magician symbolises an ability to juggle many acts at once. Need I say more! In bed he's amazing, inventive and bursting with energy. He's always on the lookout for something new and exciting, which might make him prone to straying unless you're the one keeping him on his toes.

When reversed the Magician lacks vision and has run out of steam. He's likely to make silly mistakes and then retaliate with sharp words. Generally this is caused by having given all in a previous relationship, constantly being the one to keep sex alive, and so now he's burnt out and needs time to get some bounce back into his step.

No 2 The High Priestess is all about the mysteries of life and things we don't know about. Sometimes this is simply naivety, we're inexperienced and haven't encountered anal sex or clitoral stimulation yet; let alone experienced or experimented with them. If this card represents your lover teach them slowly and gently and they'll marvel at your knowledge and experience.

This card can also represent all of the things we don't know about our lover. If it's early days of the relationship that's fine, but if we've been with our partner for some considerable time then it raises questions. Are we really that interested? If we are, and we have shown interest in their past and current life, then what are they hiding?

When reversed the High Priestess means that we do know things that we think we don't know. So, you've never given oral before, but just get down and do it, and you'll discover that you're a natural.

The High Priestess is also the card that symbolises conception. If you draw this card for the question, "How's my hot date going to go tonight?" the answer is two-fold. On the one hand it means, "Who knows?" and on the other it means "Conception." So, it's best to be on the safe side and tuck a few condoms in your pocket.

No 3 The Empress is Mother Nature and in the bedroom this translates as being your natural self. She's hot and sexy and full of life. (this applies to guys too) In fact, she's up for it. To her sex is a natural part of a loving relationship...at any age. I've seen women in their fifties and sixties draw this card and they are eager to have sex and be fulfilled.

For both men and women this is a card of great fertility, so do remember your condoms if you're not ready to start a family.

When the Empress is reversed the libido is flagging. Don't feel like it, too tired, and weird ideas about it 'not being normal' at my age...and I've heard people in their thirties spin out that phrase, believing they are past it, or on the shelf. I've even seen people in their twenties have the Empress reversed represent their sex lives. A steady relationship, work commitments and too much T.V. or computer games have sapped their sex drive and made them feel jaded before their time.

No 4 The Emperor symbolises a great sense of self worth. Sex is all a bit unadventurous, usually steady, but for a man it does represent enough stamina and self control to keep at it until his woman is satisfied. Due to their prowess this can, sometimes, lead to an element of arrogance, or bragging.

The Emperor reversed tends to be dull and a little stuffy in bed. A bit of a prude. For a man it can depict an inability to ejaculate, and for a woman difficulties in reaching a climax. Too much pride and anxiety about making noises, pulling faces and completely letting go. After all, what would your partner think if you suddenly screeched your delight or grunted your pleasure? And what if the neighbours heard! Nope, the Emperor reversed would prefer to remain uptight rather than face the embarrassment.

No 5 The High Priest symbolises communication at all levels. In order to have great sex with our partner we need to be able to communicate at a soul level, at a physical level, and through the vehicle of touch. Sound is also represented by the High Priest and in sex and romance the sound of our lover's voice can often be one of the biggest turn-ons. It's not always what they say, but the timbre of their voice that makes us go gooey.

When the High Priest is reversed that all important communication has broken down. We no longer listen, we no longer connect, and we no longer get goose-pimples up the spine when we hear their voice. This brings in another side of the High Priest, the person who listens to us; and most often these days we don't go trundling off to our priest for advice and counsel, but phone our favourite therapist. When upright it's a good and trusted therapist, but when reversed one should be wary as they usually have their own agenda and aren't able to act as a clear channel for healing and helping. Perhaps that is because you are sleeping with them, or, when we see the High Priest next to the Seven of Cups, fantasising about them in a dreamy, sexual manner.

The High Priest can also symbolise using music as a sexual stimulant.

No 6 The Lovers card does not symbolise the lover, as many people assume. No, it's a card of decision making, and the love of truth and correct choice in life. However, if we interpret the card specifically towards sex then it may represent the choice between two lovers, but more often it's all about the decision of whether or not to take a lover. For the sexual act itself it can be deciding on whether to go ahead and try things that we've never done before.

When the Lovers card is reversed no decision is made. If you're asking a question about whether someone will be your lover and this card is turned up then it means that they haven't made up their mind yet.

The Lovers card also symbolises a stage of growing up and having to make your own decisions in life, so at times it can represent an inexperienced lover, whose age belies their naivety. In general we do not anticipate luring someone in their thirties or forties into our bed only to find that they are a virgin and have no practical experience whatsoever.

No 7 The Chariot symbolises the way forwards in life and the most modern interpretation is...you've guessed it...the motor car. Yep, cars can be sexy. They add to our sex appeal. Are we a fast red Ferrari or a cute and cuddly 2CV? Surrounding cards will suggest the type of car. The Chariot can also mean that you like to have sex in a car (not so easy these days with so many cameras around) and that the open road symbolises freedom and an ability to travel to visit your lover. Long distance relationships are a possibility with this card too.

The Chariot reversed means that the relationship has gone off track and one party is no longer interested in making the effort. Sex can be a bit of a chore and unsatisfactory. Quite simply, it's going nowhere.

No 8 The Justice card shows that we have met the right person at the right time and that everything is running smoothly. Emotionally exciting on the bliss level, but not always so thrilling in bed. I've often seen this card more associated with the heart than the naughty bits, and sometimes people even say that the emotions are there but not always the sexual compatibility.

When reversed the Justice card symbolises resentment and bitterness, either in your current relationship or old stuff dragging on from previous encounters. If this is your current relationship then something is terribly wrong in bed. Does he ejaculate too quickly and leave you hungry for more? Do you spend all of your time and effort pleasing her and then she rolls over and won't let you finish? It's all unfair, unsatisfactory and leaves a bitter taste.

No 9 The Hermit is prone to secretiveness. Initially we want to be mysterious and seductive, but after a while we need to open up and share our lives. Upright this card depicts a natural, healthy caution when first meeting someone; and a desire to take things one step at a time. For sex itself the Hermit is slow, so likely to satisfy at a physical level even if he doesn't share his innermost thoughts and feelings.

When reversed the Hermit spells trouble. He is extremely closed and likely to be lying by omission. I see this card so often when someone's husband or wife is having an affair. Where have they been? What have they been doing? I've also seen it when my client is the one having the affair, the one who is being closed and guarded. In bed the reversed card nearly always creates upset due to lack of emotional intimacy and feelings of distrust between the couple.

With the reversed Hermit the extreme slowness of intercourse may end up being a total bore. Will they ever get round to penetration? There's an element of avoidance in the slowness, sometimes shyness, but mostly evading the moment when through the physical act one is required to permit another human being to get close to ones psyche as well as one's body.

Secretiveness is not always a bad thing and occasionally we all use it as a tool for self preservation. A variety of sexual acts are considered taboo or disgusting by many people, so it's best not to go shouting it round the office if we had anal sex the night before, or decided to swallow and not spit when giving a blow job. Masturbation is another dark secret that we tend to keep to ourselves. Very few of us greet our friends by saying, "Hey, I had a wank last night, and it was terrific." We will admit to having sex with our partner, but hardly ever to single sex. Then there are sex toys, the rabbit in the back of the closet, or the anal dildo hidden in a cabinet beside the bed. We'll sit with a friend and shop online for clothes, shoes, cars or motorbikes, but the 'adult shop' we visit in private.

Prostitutes are also a well kept secret, and very few men (or women) will admit to having paid for sex from a professional.

No 10 The Wheel of Fortune represents an ongoing situation, so it's likely to depict your regular partner, or that a new relationship will continue. For sex it's same old, same old, but at least it's consistent, and available, and not likely to run away.

When the Wheel of Fortune is reversed everything spins by so quickly that it's over and done with in a second. Premature ejaculation is highly likely, or the woman is trying to get it over and done with as quickly as possible. A young woman told me once that she could make any man cum in two minutes. When I asked why she even bothered her answer was simply that, "It got the sex out of the way."

No 11 The Strength card depicts self restraint, so not much sex going on here at all. Often people are brought up to be 'self controlled' and not to rush into things, but they end up never leaping into the moment, and end up missing out on the best shag of their lives. This card nearly always creates remorse in later life for all of those wonderful missed opportunities. He/she was beautiful, and I could have, but I didn't.

The Strength card reversed is a daredevil release, a breaking away and taking a risk on life. This is a card of passion and of throwing caution to the wind. When someone has had an affair they very often say, 'it just happened,' and I bet Strength reversed had something to do with it. Here we're past the thinking stage and our genitals have taken over. The heart is pounding with excitement, an adrenaline rush of intoxication takes over, and only physical satisfaction will suffice. It's exhilarating.

It need not be an affair that stimulates this card into action, but there is a boundary that is being crossed, a taboo that is being broken; whether it is one programmed in by our parents or one created by society. We are taught to wait until marriage, not to have sex on a first date, wait for the man to initiate etc. etc.. The only problem with this extreme of passion is that in the heat of the heady sexual moment we might be in too much of a rush to use a condom.

There's always haste and speed associated with Strength reversed, so if you draw this card to represent your new lover, beware, because he or she may be passionate, but fail to arouse you fully if you're not getting turned on at the same speed they are.

No 12 The Hanged Man is always waiting for something to happen, hanging around pondering life; so no sex taking place here I'm afraid. If sex does take place they are very patient and tolerant, will wait for you to have fun too; but are generally lousy at initiating anything new.

When reversed the Hanged Man is ready to leap into action, so if you've been waiting for that lover to make up their mind and call you for that hot date, now is the time. If you're in a relationship then I guess the football has just finished!

When the Hanged Man appears in a woman's reading next to the Seven of Batons, (visual stimulation) and the Ace of Batons reversed it means that she likes to look at the man's dangly bits. She gets excited watching her man cross the room naked, even when his penis is flaccid.

No 13 The Death card does not mean that you're into necrophilia...well, let's put it this way, no client of mine has ever admitted to that! It can mean the end of a relationship, it can mean a hormonal change; such as menopause; or for men, lack of libido; but in general it goes hand in glove with the Nine of Swords...the ultimate orgasm. We're back to Le Petit Mort and that blissful moment of delightful unity.

When reversed the Death card shows that we cannot let go and experience an orgasm. We are frightened of dying, and merging and blending with our lover. We are frightened of being overwhelmed and letting our body release for fear that we might truly die and never return. We might lock into the other person forever and lose our identity, and to the ego, that is truly terrifying.

For men it is an inability to ejaculate when having intercourse, although generally they are fine when on their own masturbating.

No 14 Temperance shows that we are okay, even when we don't feel okay. This is the fake it before you make it card, so with sex we are saying, 'it was great honey,' and hoping for better next time. It is disappointing, but we don't want to express this to our lover, because we know that in time things will improve. I so often see this card when one half of a couple has been over working and their partner knows they can do better, and is biding their time until the work eases up and their partner has more energy.

Temperance reversed depicts that awful moment when the partner says, 'you didn't really enjoy it, did you?' Ooops, we've been found out, and the tears roll, and we express how we really feel, and slowly we can start to sort things out.

When seen next to the Seven of Batons (visual stimulation) it means that the man enjoys looking at a woman's hips, especially when they sway as she walks.

No 15 The Devil symbolises all of those nasty little habits we've picked up over the years. "But my last lover really enjoyed it when I did that," you complain, and your new lover keeps on saying, "But I'm not them and I like it different," and you really can't break the habit. There's no teaching this dog new tricks.

Unfortunately those nasty habits can also include lack of personal hygiene. Most uninviting.

The Devil also represents guilt, and as soon as we take guilt into the bedroom we're in trouble. Guilt for being unfaithful. Guilt for doing those things our parents told us were bad. Guilt for experiencing pleasure while our partner doesn't. Guilt for not getting it right, ejaculating too quickly, making too much noise during orgasm, etc. The list goes on and on. "Sorry, didn't mean to," is the catch phrase here, a constant pitiful apology for not being good enough.

The Devil reversed is all about breaking those inhibiting habits and releasing the guilt. Much more fun.

The really negative side of the Devil reversed is when someone has an inability to experience remorse. I've only ever seen this a couple of times, but when we're talking about sex it has to be mentioned as a cautionary note. If someone doesn't experience any form of guilt over their actions then it can make them extremely dangerous. The word sorry is not in their vocabulary. If they unconsciously hurt you during sex they think nothing of it, no apology and no promise not to do it again. Has the Devil reversed come up to represent the person your child is chatting to on the internet? Be very careful.

No 16 The Tower is the shattered ego. Well that shag didn't go very well, did it! This is disastrous. Perhaps you've been fucked then dumped. Found out that your lover is married. Been told that you're crap in bed. Found out that your lover is sleeping around. Discovery of infidelity, venereal disease, your partner is gay…the list goes on. It's a total shock. Just try and get them out of the door before you break down and cry.

When the Tower is reversed our ego is still shattered, but we're putting on a brave face and trying not to let it show. The only reason for this is that we're married or have children to think about. Any other reason and it simply isn't worth it.

No 17 The Star card symbolises letting go of old stuff. Yippeee! At long last we really have experienced an orgasm. We cry with relief and the sheer joy at having let go of our invisible boundaries and gone through to the other side, a place of bliss and pleasure.

When the Star card is reversed everything appears totally hopeless. We'll never make it. We'll never orgasm, we'll never get the person of our dreams into bed, and we'll never be loved. At least this is how we feel at the time of drawing this card. Next week it may all be different.

No 18 The Moon represents fear. Here we are frightened of experiencing our pleasures, but willing to have a go. Many, many things make us fearful of sex. We are frightened of our lover seeing us naked and being put off. We are frightened of 'not being good enough.' We are frightened of it all being over and done with in two minutes. When young we're frightened of our parents coming home and finding us at it. When older we're frightened of the kids bursting in while we're at it. When old we're frightened in case we've lost it and can't perform. These are mind made fears, and can all be overcome.

Occasionally there are real fears to contend with and this goes into the realms of the dark side of sex. If you get turned on by being frightened during sex, that's fine, if not...walk away.

When the Moon card is reversed we are frightened, yet unable to move from the spot. This is terror. If this is in a real sexual situation and you can't walk away, then scream. If it's in a mind, pre-sex situation, such as terror of penetration, then find a good therapist and work through your fears in a safe environment.

No 19 The Sun symbolises bliss, happiness and contentment. Joy! This is a wonderful card where sex is concerned. It's warm, and yummy, and so delightful you'll want to stay curled up with your lover forever.

The Sun card reversed is happiness tinged with sadness, and this too is a joyous card. It shows that someone has experienced hurt and pain, sadness and loss, yet can once again experience the pleasures of life. I've often seen this card connected to sex when someone has lost a much loved partner and has now found a new partner that they can once again enjoy intimacy with. They will never forget their old love, but they don't dwell on the loss with bitterness, in fact they often say, 'I am so lucky to have found such pleasure twice in life.'

The Sun card can also represent enjoying sex outside in the sunshine. Naturist Beaches aren't there specifically for sex, but the

Sun Card symbolises enjoying walking around nude and feeling highly comfortable in your own skin, even when with other people.

No 20 Judgement represents a eureka experience. This is the moment of climax, that wonderful sound you emit as you reach the height of ecstasy. Rising out of the dark realm of separation you join with your lover in a peak experience. Superb.

When the judgement card is reversed you miss the mark and don't hit the high note. This card reversed can create the most crushing disappointment, to be so near, yet so far. It can also depict someone who has never had an orgasm, or that your lover will be unable to fulfil your needs.

No 21 The World Card symbolises the vagina. Open and inviting and ready for action. When next to the Ace of Cups the juices are flowing, so read this combination as having a healthy sexual appetite and being sexually healthy.

The World also suggests the possibility of foreign lovers and having sex while overseas or far from home.

The World card reversed depicts the closed vagina and the woman experiencing difficulties with penetration. The cause may be mental, physical or emotional, so if the problem persists it's best to visit your G.P.

It can also mean not getting out enough in order to find a lover. I see this interpretation very often for busy career minded individuals, who'd love to have sex, but never go out socially so that they can meet someone and form a relationship, or even have a one night stand.

If you're in a relationship it can mean that the relationship is all about staying at home, and you know what, after a while that can begin to make the sex life very dull and uninspiring.

Card Combinations and Practical Examples.

In tarot every card is changed by surrounding cards, so as a reader I rarely interpret one card on its own, unless I have asked my client to draw one card to see what their lover is like. However, I am more likely to ask them to draw two or three cards, so that we create a rounder picture and gain more insight.

This book would probably go on forever, and never get finished, if I tried to outline every combination of three cards, so I'll outline a few scenarios and the types of issues that clients bring to my table.

I've been a tarot reader, and astrologer, for nearly 30 years. Overall probably about 75% of my clients are women, 25% male and within the whole possibly 20% are gay (male and female); at a rough guess. I never see a client under 16 without parental/adult guidance, and so if I include younger people with a guardian present I have seen clients from aged 12 to about 90. I have read for people from most walks of life, from the very poor to the very wealthy. This gives me a pretty good cross section to draw real life material from. Work and love are the main issues raised, and sometimes a client will be refreshingly honest and admit outright that their quest is for sex, as well as relationship.

Infidelity

The Page of Cups reversed symbolises unfaithfulness, disloyalty and being fed up with serving others.

Each person is different in what they believe to be unfaithfulness, or infidelity, in a relationship. In Western culture we expect, or anticipate, exclusivity, especially in sexual matters. However, emotional intimacy with someone outside the relationship can be as equally damaging as sex outside the relationship. For some individuals infidelity is the fact that their partner doesn't come home straight after work and prefers to spend time with someone of the opposite sex, just 'having a coffee,' but in truth is giving this other person much more of their personal time and attention. Very often this type of extra marital friendship, strays, meanders, or plunges into a sexual encounter; even though it appears to have started innocently enough. For other people unfaithfulness is the sex act itself, and conversation doesn't count, the final, intimate boundary of the physical body the ultimate digression. I had one client, who on discovering that his long term partner was having an affair said, "It isn't the sex, it's the deceit."

So we see that unfaithfulness is always how the partner being hurt experiences the situation. It's about a lack of faithfulness and loyalty. If the couple don't talk through issues any more, then one partner snuggling up to someone else over coffee and sharing their problems, is a total slap in the face.

In Tarot the Page of Cups upright is loyal and faithful. He (or she) enjoys being there for their partner and doing things for them as well as with them. It isn't sacrificial, it's consideration and tenderness. When the Page of Cups is reversed he simply can't be bothered any more, or does things for his partner in a half hearted, resentful fashion. That is when he hooks up with someone who appears to demand less, and stops considering his partner's needs.

Let's look at a few combinations of the Page of Cups reversed alongside other cards.

As I mentioned earlier the sequence the cards are turned in is very important. If we look at the Page of Cups reversed next to the Queen of Swords we can see two distinct pictures.

Queen of Swords first, Page of Cups reversed second would suggest that the wife (female partner) is having gynaecological problems, possibly has just given birth, or is menstruating. This has temporarily made her a non-sexual being because she is physically 'unavailable.' It also means that she will require more care and attention, more tolerance because her hormones are making her irritable, and an element of consideration that some may consider 'hard work.' This natural, but testing situation, then makes the male partner go and look for sexual satisfaction outside the relationship.

Page of Cups reversed first and Queen of Swords second. The Page of Cups is naturally a very caring individual. If his partner appears to be 'capable' then he will often go looking for 'the bird with the broken wing,' someone who is having a hard time and needs his time and attention. The Queen of Swords is the widowed, divorced or separated woman, so suddenly we have the perfect hook, a woman in distress who needs him. Often the Queen of Swords will lure him, but sometimes she acts unconsciously, her need for a replacement man, who isn't necessarily seeking commitment, the perfect solution. When they meet she isn't ready to commit either, hence she can feel comfortable. She will simply borrow someone else's partner for a while until she feels better.

Next to the Six of Cups (both upright and reversed) the Page of Cups reversed is lured away by somebody from their past. You wouldn't believe how many times I saw this combination when Friends Reunited first took off. Dozens of people sat at my table openly admitting that they had secretly visited an old flame from school days, tracked down their lost love, or slept with the guy they should have married. Only when we see the Knight of Cups next to these two cards does the person actually take off to be with their lover, to see where it might go, or, having tasted divine love again, decide to leave their regular relationship anyway.

If we're talking about a straight forward sexual encounter, with no hidden agenda, then the Page of Cups reversed will appear next to the Ace of Batons or the Strength card reversed. Hot blooded passion reared its head, and if you ask them why they did it they'll simply say they couldn't help themselves.

Jealousy

The Three of Swords symbolises jealousy, as well as anger. It is destructive, whether you are on the receiving end or experiencing it.

Here are some examples of the jealous side of the **Three of Swords** next to various cards.

The Queen of Batons – For women, your lover is seen with someone you think is prettier than you.

The Four of Coins – Someone is wealthier than you.

The Nine of Coins reversed – You feel abandoned in favour of a best mate/favourite sport/computer game/work – innocent pastimes that give your partner pleasure.

The Queen of Swords – For women it's your monthly and you're full of p.m.t. This combination can also be seen after childbirth and during menopause. It's hormonal. Basically you're out of action and can end up grumpy and jealous even if he pays your pet more attention.

Three of Cups – Your lover is married and has to return to their husband/wife. Hey! How come they are getting all of the 'quality' days, such as Christmas and Bank Holidays? Or even your birthday.

Ten of Coins – Family jealousies... which can easily interfere with the best of relationships.

Five of Coins reversed – You feel unsupported, and believe that others get more help than you. "But you cooked your best mate dinner, so why won't you do that for me?"

Ace of Swords reversed – You've been lied to. Yes, he/she did sleep with their ex, and swore blind that they didn't when you asked them last week. They probably lied about using a condom as well.

The Hermit reversed– Far too many secrets that create suspicion.

The Six of Coins reversed – They got what they wanted and didn't bother about you.

The seven of Cups – Sorry, but it's all in your imagination.

The Dating Game

Before it all goes belly up we've usually experienced the halcyon days, or what most people call 'the honeymoon period.' Whether married, just getting together, or having some fun, there is always that exciting and joyful first few days, or months, which we later look back upon with wistful desire.

Let's look at the dating game and finding that perfect partner who will sexually delight us for years.

What I see for many clients is that they are going out looking for a partner in the wrong place. If you're a serious type and you go out with your mates to the local night club then it's very likely that you'll end up with the wrong type of person.

Let's look at some examples of going out and trying to attract a partner from the viewpoint of a young single female.

Miss **Queen of Cups** is looking for tenderness and someone she can slightly mother. On a bad night she's very likely to fall for a lame dog in the guise of Mr Page of Swords who is cocky, self assured and likely to prey on her sweet nature. In bed she will look to please him and be disappointed when he doesn't phone afterwards, not understanding that it was a fling, and that he didn't mean all of those sweet words he said last night.

If she connects with Mr King of Coins she'll be thrilled by the quality of the meal on offer, the expertise of his sexual performance; but be disappointed if they become involved in a long term relationship because he'll end up treating her like a possession and constantly be out working. In some circumstances this can suit Miss Queen of Cups, because she adores family and children, and likes to be looked after.

Miss **Queen of Batons** is looking for some sex. She's fun and enjoys excitement and the chase. She'll recognise Mr Page of Swords for what he is and either go along for the ride or not bother getting involved.

She's likely to have most fun with Mr King of Batons, because they will be well suited sexually and have fun together. Mostly she will find Mr King of Coins too inhibiting, and as for Mr King of Cups, well initially she might be attracted, but in general she'll find him a bit of a push over and not a strong enough type.

Miss **Queen of Coins** is always looking for quality, so she'll be attracted to Mr King of Coins, enjoy everything on offer and continue to go back for more. Occasionally she'll fall for Mr Page of Swords because he's exciting and full of promises concerning future wealth, plus he dresses to kill and can easily be mistaken for a prosperous business man. However, if she's had sex with Mr Page of Swords she may find returning to the security of the Mr King of Coins type lacking in sexual excitement and settle for second best in bed. Don't get me wrong, Mr King of Coins is a highly accomplished lover, but he's less likely to experiment with anal sex or watching pornography together.

Miss **Queen of Swords** is only likely to go out looking for sex if she's widowed or divorced, the other side of her which has gynaecological issues just doesn't want to initiate anything. Unfortunately widowed or divorced women can sometimes act desperate when dating, and this can often make the man feel trapped or rushed, and therefore spoil the fun if all the pillow talk after sex is geared towards a long term future when it was supposed to be a casual fling. She will, of course, be prepared to sleep with any man if she's been bereft of sex for a long while and feels the years ticking by.

Now let's look at a few examples for men going out looking for sex and fun.

Mr **King of Cups** is likely to feel lost out on the dating field. He likes to be intimate on a one-to-one basis, share a meal and find out about his potential new lover before jumping into bed. He does better at social clubs and societies than night clubs and pubs. He's more likely to chat up the girl he fancies in the corner shop than go out especially looking for sex.

Mr **King of Batons** loves life to the full so he'll be darting backwards and forwards to the gym, busy travelling, and hooking up with his mates to go out for a boys' night out to find some girls. Shy Mr King of Cups might well be one of the friends he's dragged along, and there's generally a Mr Page of Swords somewhere in his circle of friends, after all, he will accept everyone as his friend.

He'll be most attracted to a pretty girl as he's a handsome chap, so he'll go for Miss Queen of Batons or Miss Queen of Cups. Both can give him a good time, although for a longer relationship he's likely to choose the gentler Miss Queen of Cups, who can tame some of his wild side, and will spend hours massaging much more than his ego.

Mr **King of Coins** acts in pretty much the same way as his female counterpart, preferring a quality match and someone he feels he can trust once he's invested time and effort. He isn't mercenary, but does anticipate a payoff. So if he pays for any woman to have a meal, he will expect sex. He may well be attracted to Miss Queen of Swords, especially if she's widowed, because she has a good track record, stayed with her husband and is probably well set up financially and therefore won't be too expensive to run. She also has a wealth of sexual experience which means they can get on with quality sex right from the start without him needing to waste time training anyone up.

The other side of Mr King of Coins enjoys moulding a fresh young Page of Batons into precisely what he is looking for sexually in a woman. This combination is very often the older man with a much younger woman.

Mr **King of Swords**…well he's usually got other things to think about than sex, so hardly ever goes out looking for it. If he does then he'll moan and be discontent because he is seeking perfection, and you hardly ever get that the first time you sleep with a new partner. He'll also lay down the law and tell the woman precisely what he wants, so absolutely no lee way for experimentation; and definitely no laughing.

These are just a few examples and obviously there are loads of other combinations, because people will be shown as one person when at home, different while out, and different yet again when looking for sex.

Final Thoughts

There are probably some sexual issues I haven't covered in this volume and that is most likely because I haven't specifically seen it mentioned during a tarot reading. One question I've been wracking my brains over is "Which card, or card combination, symbolises anal sex?" I've read for loads of gay men, and women who enjoy anal sex, but the cards have never specified the act itself. Generally it's been hinted at through our complex friend the Page of Swords, who's up for anything sexually; and very often coupled with the Hermit reversed, showing that it's a taboo subject that's being indulged in.

Stimulation via spanking is another one covered by the Page of Swords, but the degree of pain administered is difficult to determine because the card alongside it is often the Nine of Swords, which also depicts brutal sex in this combination. One of my clients used to turn up with bruises all over her because her husband was so rough, and in her instance it was an unhealthy, perverse act that he was getting his jollies from and making her very unhappy.

Blissful sex is easy to see in the cards. The Ace of Batons alongside the Two of Cups and Judgement, is near enough a perfect combination. Sex, love and orgasm.

However you like your sex continue to enjoy it and follow your bliss. Do whatever turns you on as long as it doesn't harm anyone else. Sex is a natural part of life and brings us joy, happiness and a special closeness to another human being.

Printed in Great Britain
by Amazon